# Yoga for the Young at Heart

## Gentle Stretching Exercises for Seniors

GENTLE
STRETCHING
EXERCISES FOR SENIORS

# YOGA for the YO

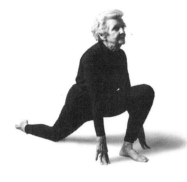

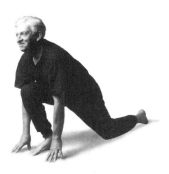

# NG
## at HEART

### SUSAN WINTER WARD
#### PHOTOGRAPHY BY JOHN SIROIS

CAPRA PRESS
SANTA BARBARA

Cover design, book design, typography and image scanning
by Frank Goad, Santa Barbara, California

Film by In Color, Santa Barbara, California


LIBRARY OF CONGRESS CATALOGING-IN-PUBLICATION DATA

Ward, Susan Winter
Yoga for the young at heart  :  gentle flow yoga for seniors  /  Susan Winter Ward :
photography by John Sirois.
p.    cm.
ISBN 0-88496-376-4 ( pbk. )  :  $12.95
1.  Yoga , Hatha.   2.  Aged--Health  and  hygiene.
I.  Title.
RA781.7.W37   1994
613.7'046--dc20                                93-42586
CIP


CAPRA PRESS
Post Office Box 2068
Santa Barbara, CA 93120

*To my father, Carl,*
*and my mother, Julia,*
*who both taught me about*
*love, confidence, patience and trust.*

# ACKNOWLEDGMENTS

YOGA HAS CHANGED MY LIFE. When I took my first class, I definitely was not enthralled, but I heard a little voice inside me say, "You don't have to like it, just do it." Experience has taught me to listen to that voice. After my third Yoga class I was hooked, and my body and soul have never been the same. The experience keeps unfolding in surprising ways. The existence of this book is a perfect example.

This book seems to have been guided into reality. I never set out to write a Yoga book; all the pieces necessary for its creation just appeared at the right time. I deeply appreciate the privilege of being the one to bring it together, and acknowledge with heartfelt gratitude all those who have participated in bringing it to life:

My dear friend Starlina Riparetti, who dragged me to my first Yoga class; Ganga White and Tracey Rich, who have provided the teaching and inspiration, the Flow Series and White Lotus retreats; my dedicated senior Yoga students at the Samarkand in Santa Barbara; my mother, Julia Winter Cohen, for her constant encouragement, support and love; "my Sis," Maggie Sanders, the Colonel's daughter, for giving me the pep talk to get this ball rolling; Noel Young, for his vote of confidence and willingness to publish my first book; Joel Block, who held my hand through the early stages of writing and continues in his encouragement; and Dr. Donald O. Fareed for orthopedic expertise and suggestions.

This book wouldn't be complete without the photographic abilities and patience of John Sirois. Somehow we always connect at special times in our lives to help each other. Deep appreciation also goes to the splendid subjects of John's photography, Babs Raymond and Otto Mortensen, who both spent hours cheerfully posing for the camera.

Through this co-creative spirit, this book nows gives you the opportunity to explore a new way of being in your body. It was written for you. May you use it in good health and enjoy the process of self-discovery.

# ~ CONTENTS ~

# ⚡ FOREWORD ⚡

Y OGA HAS BEEN A GIFT in our lives—one of the greatest gifts we have ever given ourselves. It has brought grace, strength and flexibility to our bodies and allowed us to have greater agility in sports and our pursuits in nature. Even more, Yoga has become a way of being, a way of seeing and, if you will, a way of life.

In our years of being both students and teachers of Yoga we have witnessed exceptional transformations in people: some ever so subtle, some quite profound. It is no wonder Yoga has been considered mysterious or dubbed "the elixir of youth" because its ability to restore the body and support the "life force" seems almost magical. But in reality it is scientific too, and it begins with the first breath.

Most of us have never been trained to breathe properly. We consider it part of the package we came with. Perhaps it is, but sitting in chairs and cars all day, living in congested cities or watching the Dow rise and fall, is not. These things disturb our breathing, our bodies and our perspectives. Learning how to breathe properly, to sit, to stand and walk, in essence to live comfortably, are areas addressed in Yoga and in this book.

The Flow Series, on which this book is based, was developed as a balanced daily workout. It uses the classical poses and breath work of Hatha Yoga and is designed as a moving meditation. The Flow Series combines body movements and breathing in synchronicity, creating strength and stamina, skeletal and muscular alignment, cardiovascular health, flexibility and mental clarity. Allowing the mind to float upon the breath and the body to flow into the positions brings one increased vitality and creates a meditative state which can flow into daily life.

Susan Ward's keen appreciation of Yoga is apparent in her adaptation of the Flow Series, a practice designed especially for our older citizens. She has strong compassion for seniors and is committed to contributing to their health and well-being. This series can be adjusted to each person's level and pace so that all you need to do is begin.

We wish you a lifetime of living comfortably with your body and spirit.

*Namaste,*
TRACEY RICH and GANGA WHITE
The White Lotus Foundation
Santa Barbara, California

# ⚓ INTRODUCTION ⚓

YOGA IS AN ADVENTURE. I have been continually impressed with the changes it makes in people's bodies and lives, including my own, and welcome you to your own personal practice.

Regardless of your age or physical condition, a gentle and consistent Hatha Yoga practice can bring you significant benefits. It builds strength, increases flexibility and circulation, and teaches deep relaxation through a series of slow and gentle body poses and controlled breathing techniques which can be adapted to everyone's abilities.

This book can be your guide to developing a stronger and more vital body no matter what your physical condition may be. All you need to reap the benefits of a Yoga practice is a willingness to begin, and to be open to new ways of experiencing your body. Yoga is a process; there is no goal. It is an ongoing discovery of physical and psychological challenges met with gentleness and sensitivity through which the body may relax, open, come into balance, and become healthier.

It is important to meet your inevitable resistances with gentleness and to encourage your body to relax. Mother Teresa has said "Do no great things, but small things with great love." So love yourself, listen carefully to what your body is telling you about its limitations and respect it. In this way your Yoga practice will be both enjoyable and beneficial.

Hundreds of books have been written on Yoga and all of its attendant histories, philosophies, practices, and poses. If you want an in-depth study of more of the Yogic practices and traditions, please refer to my Bibliography and Suggested Reading. With that in mind, I have kept this book concise and to the point to create a guide for a simple personal Yoga practice specifically designed for Seniors.

Yoga need not be intimidating for anyone, no matter what their physical capacities. As Ganga White of the White Lotus Foundation says, "Begin where you are and stay there."

We will begin with the basics:

⊡ YOGA: The origins of Yoga are shrouded in the mists of time, but it is believed to have originated three to four thousand years ago in India. Over the centuries, many theories, philosophies, and systems have developed as expressions of personal, physical, spiritual and mystical quests.

Today, Yoga classes of many different types and systems are popping up everywhere. Yoga classes stressing fitness feature as many different styles of teaching Yoga as there are teachers. The general term for "physical fitness Yoga" is "Hatha" Yoga.

⊡ HATHA YOGA: The word "Hatha" (pronounced HA-tah) comes from the Sanskrit "Ha" meaning sun and "Tha" meaning moon. "Hatha," therefore, expresses the balance of opposing forces, sun-moon, male-female, positive-negative, and so on. "Yoga" means union or reintegration. So in "Hatha Yoga" we have the union or reintegration of opposing forces. Through Yoga, the mind and body can reintegrate and restore balance. Buddha said, "To keep the body in good health is a duty, otherwise we shall not be able to keep our mind strong and clear." If our body and mind are balanced, strong and clear, all other aspects of our world are open to us.

⊡ FLOW YOGA: The concept of "flow" in Yoga is called "vinyasa" and relates to the linking of one pose to the next and to the next and so on and so on. Ganga White and Tracey Rich of the White Lotus Foundation in Santa Barbara, California, have developed the Flow Series, a strong and challenging Yoga practice intended to build strength, flexibility, and stamina. The Yoga practice developed for Seniors in this book is an adaptation of their Flow Series. It is designed to create the same type of benefits as a more vigorous practice, yet is adapted for those with less strength and athletic ability.

The "flow" style of Yoga allows the body to flow gracefully from one pose into the next to create a peaceful, meditative movement. The series of poses in this guidebook are meant to be linked together through the body and the breath working in harmony. Rather than thinking of this practice as a set of separate poses, they are intended to be integrated from beginning to end and thought of as a continuous movement.

If the entire series seems too challenging to you, begin by holding each pose briefly, and moving slowly from one pose into the next until that process becomes easier. Hold the poses for a short time at first and gradually move toward smoothing out the transitions between poses and increasing your "holding time."

⊡ DEDICATION: We all have heard that practice makes perfect, but in the case of a Yoga practice, there is no perfection. The more consistent the practice, however, the more quickly the results are evident. I've heard many new Yoga students enthusiastically report that they felt relaxed, energized, and an inch taller after their first

Yoga class. Everyone's first Yoga experience is a personal one, and the feelings and effects vary as one's practice unfolds. The results become more refined and subtle over time. A Yoga practice is an ever-changing experience. Remember, today's practice will be different from tomorrow's, your right side is different from your left, and your body changes from one moment to the next. Constant openmindedness and allowing your body to be just the way it is at each moment will create an atmosphere of relaxation and acceptance in every moment of your practice.

Begin slowly. You will discover how many hours a week feels right for you. Consistency is important. It is better to do a half hour of Yoga every day than two hours once a week. A balanced practice for one person may be one and a half hours every other day, for another it may be a half hour every day. You don't need to be rigid, but be consistent. If you tune in and listen to your body it will tell you what feels appropriate.

It also helps to note benchmarks of progression in your practice. For example, make a mental note that your hands come just below your knees in a Forward Fold. Several weeks later you may notice that your hands come to center of your shin. It is exciting to be able to look back and see where you've been.

⊡ ATTITUDE: Hatha Yoga requires that you be ultimately responsible for your own health. Stiffness, poor circulation, digestive problems, lack of physical strength, and many other ailments, do not need to be accepted as the inevitable result of aging. A consistent practice of Yoga, along with a healthy diet and positive attitude can help relieve these and other symptoms commonly associated with the aging process. They can be replaced with increased flexibility, efficient circulation and digestion, and increased strength. Consistent Yoga brings a sense of groundedness, well-being and clarity, all of which allow life to be more dynamic and enjoyable.

Be kind and gentle with yourself. If this type of stretching and breathing is new to you, it will take time to get used to it and develop an awareness of what your body is telling you. Listen to your body, explore your limits and tensions gently. Go slowly and always respect pain. If a pose is hurting you, stop, back off to a point of a comfortable stretch, breathe, and allow your body to release slowly. Remember, there is no goal, Yoga is a lifelong learning process of personal unfoldment; it is getting to know yourself from the inside out.

How you approach your Yoga practice, your priorities, patience, and sensitivity can tell you quite a bit about how you approach life. I've found Yoga to be a microcosm of how I approach challenges, implement self-discipline, respond to discomfort, and integrate spirituality into my life. The personal lessons that we need to learn seem to be reflected in our Yoga practice.

⊡ A WORD ABOUT DIET: In caring for our bodies it is important to be aware that our bodies need nutritious and health-giving foods. Much of what is presented to us as "food" is convenient, nicely packaged and/or highly processed. It is filled with additives, preservatives and mostly devoid of nutritional value. The cumulative effects in our bodies of chemicals, toxins, stress and environmental hazards cannot be measured, and are in different combinations unique to each of us. Awareness of nutritional eating, relaxation and bringing our bodies into balance can help to cleanse us of these 20th-century hazards.

Traditionally, Yogis are vegetarians. Over the centuries they have found a vegetarian diet to be healthier and many people practicing Yoga find that eventually their taste for meat diminishes. Since there is now a body of evidence that many diseases commonly associated with aging can be prevented, improved and possibly cured by eating a diet free of animal products and fats, this dietary alteration may have beneficial long term affects. In the Suggested Reading list at the back of this book, you will find listed some of the many new books on the subject. I encourage you to explore them. The consensus is that adding lots of fresh fruits and vegetables, whole grains and seeds along with plenty of water could be an extremely valuable alteration to your diet.

⊡ BREATHING: The breath or life force is called "prana" (pronounced PRA-nah). We usually take our breathing for granted, but we obviously cannot survive for long without it. The "prana" or breath that we inhale brings oxygen and life force to every cell in our bodies. The way you breathe plays a key role in your Yoga practice. By concentrating on the rhythm of the breath, the body and the breath harmonize into a flowing, energizing experience in movement.

Coordinating the breath with body movements allows the body to move more easily and can also control the intensity of the poses. Each pose is usually held for a period of 3 to 5 breaths (a breath is a full inhalation and complete exhalation). The poses then follow one after the other with the body moving in harmony with the inhalations and exhalations.

Try this example. Sit in an armless chair and inhale as you raise your arms out to your sides and overhead, then exhale as you lower your arms down by your sides. Experiment with this movement, first breathing passively and then intentionally with your breath moving in harmony with your body. Do you feel the difference?

It may help to visualize for a moment what is actually happening when we breathe. We usually take it for granted and don't realize what a miracle each breath is. The lungs are made up of millions of tiny air sacs which handle the exchange of gases in our bodies on the cellular level, cleansing and oxygenating the body. The lungs take up a considerable amount of space in the body, actually extending from the collarbones down almost to the bottom of the rib cage.

In general, we breathe shallowly with only the top portions of our lungs. Experiment with the depth of your breathing by seeing how you can gradually bring your breath deeper into your lungs with each inhalation. Bring your breath gently into your lungs, imagining the expansion of each little air sac inside, as if you were inflating a myriad of tiny balloons.

It is also important to understand what is happening on a more visible level when we breathe. When inhaling, as the air is flowing into the lungs the diaphragm drops, the rib cage expands outward and up, and the upper chest lifts. On exhalation, the diaphragm lifts, rib cage contracts and the upper chest drops.

Although this seems elementary, a way to get acquainted with this phenomenon is to place one hand on your stomach and the other on one side of your rib cage. As you inhale feel your stomach expand and your rib cage move outward. As you exhale, feel the contraction. Try this for a few breaths with your eyes closed to really experience what happens in your body when you breathe.

In order to keep awareness on the breath, Yoga practice uses a technique called "Ujjayi" (pronounced "oo-jai-ee") meaning "victorious." Using this technique, a sound is created similar to the sound of breathing through Scuba equipment, a snorkel or a throaty snore. The sounds of inhalation and exhalation become audible so that it is easier to stay aware of your breath throughout the practice.

It can take a little practice to learn to make your breathing audible. The Ujjayi sound of the breath comes from the soft palate at the back of the throat, almost like a purr or whisper. To learn this breathing technique whisper the word "whisper," prolonging the "perrrr" part as you inhale and exhale through your mouth several times. Concentrate on where the sound is coming from and continue the sound as you close your mouth and breathe through your nose. While practicing Yoga, breathe only through your nose. As the Yogis say, "The mouth is for eating, the nose is for breathing." Try to keep your inhalations and exhalations of equal duration as you relax and listen to the sound of your breath. It may seem strange and awkward at first, but with just a little practice it will soon become a natural part of your Yoga practice.

Breathing keeps your energy flowing throughout your body. Holding your breath blocks that flow. If a pose is challenging, breathe. Focus on steady inhalation and exhalations. Listen to your breath.

⊡ RELAXATION: Allowing your body to ease into a pose is the key to a pleasant and effective Yoga experience. If the body is pushed too far too fast it will resist, as most of us do psychologically as well. If one has a mental concept of what the body "should" do and pushes it to achieve that concept, it is likely the body will experience tension, pain and even injury.

Relax. Our bodies respond well to coaxing. If a pose initially seems too challenging, back away from the edge of your resistance, concentrate on your deep breathing and relax into the pose. It's surprising how the body responds to the release of tension through the relaxing sound of the breath. You will notice that the poses are active, not static, and that as your body releases you can take the stretches a little farther. The next time you do the same pose, you will notice how much more easily your body will be gently nudged into the stretch.

Another aspect of relaxation in Yoga practice is called "savasana" and is considered by many to be the "big payoff." At the end of your Yoga session, it is extremely important to allow your body to relax and integrate the benefits of your practice, and is also very pleasurable, so don't miss it!

At the end of each session lie quietly on your back releasing your body weight to the floor. Take several long, deep, slow inhalations and exhalations and then allow your body to resume its natural breathing rhythm. Release all tension. It can help to visualize releasing tightness from your feet, your ankles, your calves, knees, and so on up through your body to the crown of your head. Allow yourself to completely relax for at least five minutes. It's fine to fall asleep. You will arise from this deep relaxation with a renewed sense of well-being.

⊡ **WHERE AND WHEN:** Yoga time is your time, especially for yourself. Eliminate interruptions, unplug the telephone, turn off the TV, put the cat out, and try to clear your space of distractions. Yoga requires us to be attentive to our bodies and our breath. It helps to have a protective attitude about creating this time and space for yourself.

The best environment for Yoga is one which is clean, free from drafts, and spacious enough for your body to move freely. A firm, non-slippery floor surface like hardwood or a non-plushy carpet are preferable. Many people use a mat. If you do, be sure it is firm and used on a hard floor.

Wear comfortable clothes that will easily move with your body. Avoid clothes that bunch up or are oversized. Dance tights, cotton pants or shorts are fine.

Yoga should be done barefooted. Socks allow your feet to slip around inside of them and shoes interfere with the natural movement of the muscles of your feet. Give your body a break from restrictions—physical and mental!

Yoga is best on an empty stomach. If you choose to do your practice during the day or in the evening be sure to put two or more hours between your food and your "forward fold."

Choose a time of day that works for you, when you won't feel rushed or out of sorts. Some people rise at six A.M. full of vitality and others don't come alive until ten o'clock at night. Although Yoga can certainly get you going in the morning and relax you at night, let your body and your biological clock be your guide. The important thing is to be consistent in your dedication to yourself.

⊡ A CAUTIONARY NOTE: If you have any question as to the suitability of this practice for you or have any serious physical problems, have had recent surgery or are suffering from glaucoma, high blood pressure, or hypertension, please consult with your physician before beginning this or any other exercise practice. It is especially important to check on the suitability of poses that require you to bend over forward or lower your head below your heart.

⊡ REASSURANCES: Whenever we try something new and different, it's natural to feel both psychological and physical resistance. Sometimes we begin a new experience or commitment with a burst of energy which soon fizzles. Yoga, however, is its own reward. Almost immediately, the body responds to the cleansing and oxygenating benefits of deep rhythmic breathing, and to the balancing and increased efficiency of all the body's systems through the gentle stretching and relaxing into the poses. Be forewarned: Yoga can be addictive. The body, mind and soul love it!

Muscles which have been half asleep for years are about to be roused from their slumber and are bound to reawaken slowly. If you experience sore or aching muscles a hot tub and/or gentle massage may help. Usually stretching the sore area very gently will bring relief.

There is a difference between pain and muscle soreness, and it is important to tune into your body to distinguish between them. Pain is telling you that something is definitely wrong, you're pushing too hard or your body is out of alignment. Pain is your body's way of telling you to stop immediately.

Aching muscles are telling you that something is right! You can feel the stretch of resistant places in your body and you're challenging your body to become more flexible, stronger and more vital. As you progress with your practice your body may go through a process of realignment. Try not to let preliminary discomforts discourage you. The sure cure for them is to stay with a consistent Yoga practice.

Don't be surprised if you feel new things happening in your body. It will be making changes as you progress in your practice. You are bound to feel different sensations as your body becomes more flexible, stronger, more relaxed and your internal organs and systems come into balance.

Let's begin.

# WELCOME
# TO YOUR
# YOGA
# PRACTICE

# POSE 1: STANDING MOUNTAIN POSE

*"The important thing is this, to be able to sacrifice at
any moment what we are for what we could become."*
—Chas DuBois

⊡ Stand with the balls of your feet together and your heels slightly apart, arms relaxed at your sides.

⊡ Feel your weight evenly distributed on both feet.

⊡ Press your feet into the floor as you lift through the crown of your head.

⊡ Tuck your tailbone under slightly and lift your lower ribs away from the top of your hips bones.

⊡ Lift your chest as you inhale deeply, relaxing your shoulders back and down. Begin your "Ujjayi" or audible breathing.

⊡ Continue deep inhalations and complete exhalations listening to the sound of your breath. Take 5 to 10 deep, complete breaths.

⊡ As you breathe, continue to press your body below the waist toward the floor and lift your body above the waist toward the ceiling. Maintain the lift even as you exhale.

⊡ As you inhale . . .

BENEFITS: Aligns body posture, evenly distributes weight on both feet, improves balance, brings a sense of alertness and poise.

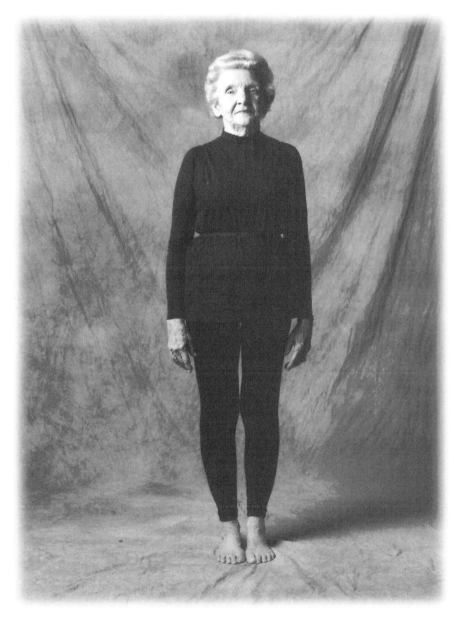

# ⇁ POSE 2: ARMS OVERHEAD ⇀

*"The great thing in this world is not so much where*
*we are, but in what direction we are moving."*
—Oliver Wendell Holmes

⊡ Raise your arms out to your sides and up overhead, palms facing each other.

⊡ As you lift, imagine pulling energy up through your feet. Bring the energy up through your body and let it flow out of your fingertips.

⊡ As you inhale feel your ribs expand and separate as you lengthen your waist.

⊡ Try to maintain the lift as you exhale and stretch your fingertips toward the ceiling. Keeping your shoulders relaxed back and down.

⊡ Keep your body active, lifting and expanding as you take 3 to 5 breaths.

⊡ Take a deep inhalation and . . .

BENEFITS: Exercises the lungs, strengthens the muscles of the arms, shoulders, chest, and back.

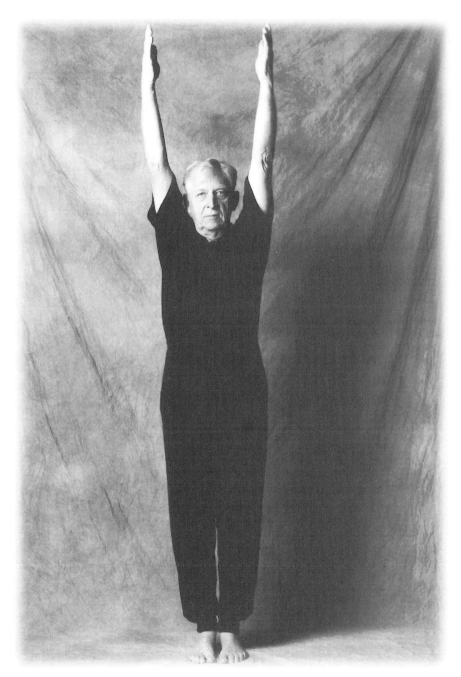

*"The chiefest point of happiness,
that a man is willing to be what he is."*
—Desiderius Erasmus (1465-1536)

⊞ Exhale as you slowly lower your arms down to your sides and clasp them behind you.

⊞ Inhale deeply, then exhale completely as you press your knuckles toward the floor.

⊞ As you inhale keep your chin tucked in, expanding and lifting your chest.

⊞ As you exhale, press gently out the back of your neck, keeping your tailbone tucked slightly under.

⊞ Continue your deep breathing for 3 to 5 breaths, then . . .

BENEFITS: Opens the chest, stretches and relaxes the shoulders.

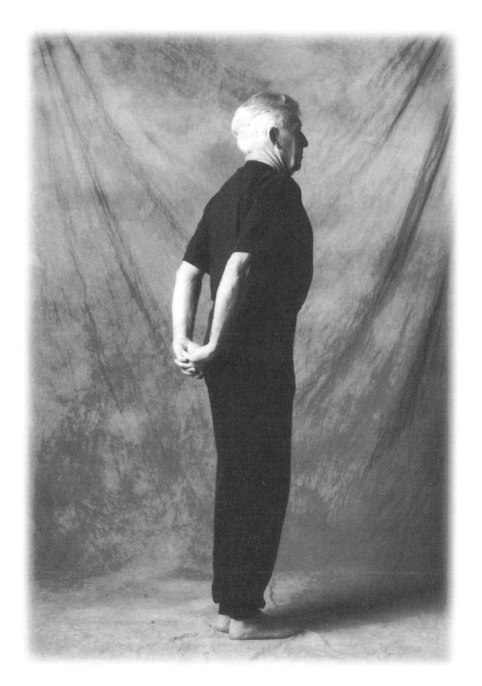

# POSE 4: NECK STRETCHES

*"Whatever you can do, or dream you can, begin it.*
*Boldness has genius, power and magic in it."*
—Goethe

Forward stretch:

⊡ With your hands still clasped behind you, tuck your chin toward the soft spot of your throat.

⊡ Inhale as you bring your chin and your chest toward each other. Keep pressing the palms of your hands together and your knuckles toward the floor.

⊡ As you exhale allow the weight of your head to gently stretch the back of your neck.

⊡ Relax into the stretch as you take 3 to 5 breaths.

BENEFITS: Releases muscle tension in the back of the neck and upper back between the shoulder blades. Opens the chest and stretches the shoulders. Strengthens breathing.

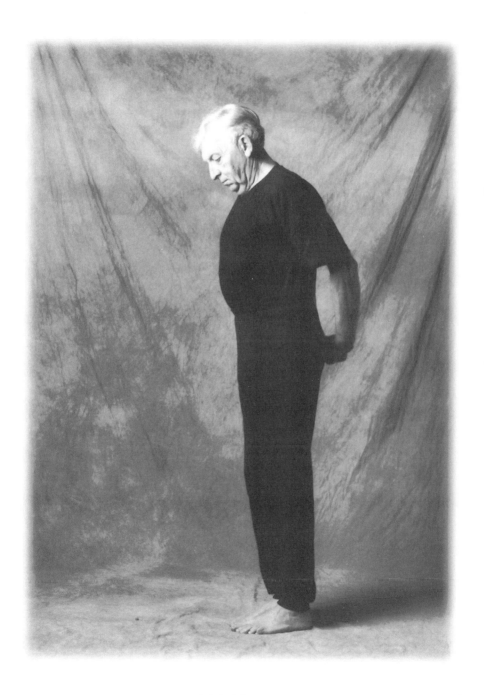

**Side stretches:**
Release your hands and allow your arms to be relaxed at your sides.

**Right Side:**

⊡ Keeping your chin tucked in, take a long, slow inhalation.

⊡ Exhale as you tip your right ear toward your right shoulder (The ear goes toward the shoulder, not the shoulder toward the ear).

⊡ Keep your shoulders relaxed and gently press your left shoulder down as you exhale, releasing the left side of your neck.

**Left Side:**

⊡ Keep your chin tucked in toward your throat.

⊡ Repeat the stretch on the other side bringing your left ear toward your left shoulder, pressing down the right shoulder as you exhale, stretching the right side of your neck.

⊡ Remember to breathe deeply and give an equal number of breaths to each side.

BENEFITS: Stretches and releases the sides of the neck and tops of the shoulders, strengthens the neck muscles.

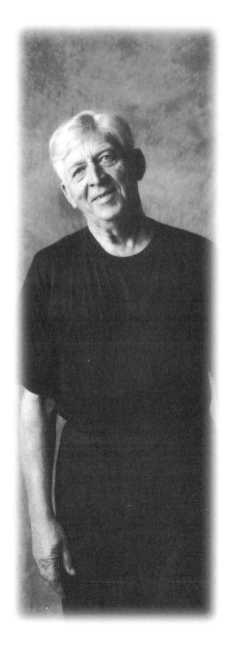
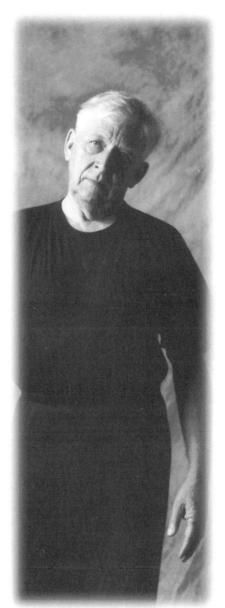

# POSE 5: ARMS OVERHEAD

*"One can never consent to creep when one*
*feels an impulse to soar."*
—Helen Keller

⊡ Take a long slow inhalation as you raise your arms out to the sides and overhead.

⊡ Lift through your fingertips and press into the floor with your feet.

⊡ Feel space being created between your ribs as you inhale.

⊡ Maintain the lift as you exhale slowly.

⊡ Take 3 to 5 breaths, then a deep inhalation as you . . .

BENEFITS: Stretches and tones the arm muscles, chest, shoulders, back and abdomen. Strengthens posture and balance.

Optional Poses (A) TREE and (B) TRIANGLE may be inserted here. See pages 92 and 94.

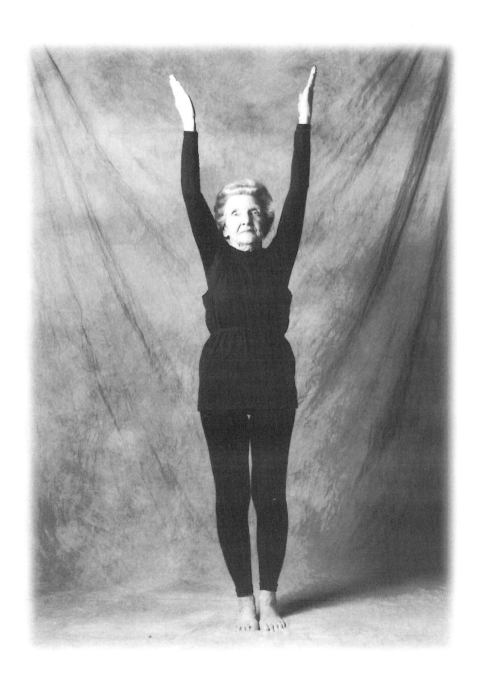

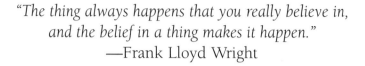
*"The thing always happens that you really believe in,*
*and the belief in a thing makes it happen."*
—Frank Lloyd Wright

⊡ Reach out through your fingertips as you fold forward, exhaling slowly.

⊡ As you come forward, keep your back flat as long as you comfortably can, then round over forward continuing to roll down one vertebrae at a time.

⊡ If you need to take several breaths, pause in your downward motion as you inhale and then continue to roll down as you exhale.

⊡ At the bottom of your forward fold let your arms dangle toward the floor.

⊡ Relax your neck and your head.

⊡ Gently bring your breath as deeply into your lungs as possible and exhale completely. Take 3 to 5 breaths, then . . .

OPTIONS: Weak Lower Back: If the pose seems too challenging for you, you may want to experiment with some of these variations:
• 1. Bring your arms out to your sides, shoulder height, rather than overhead.
• 2. Let your arms relax at your sides and roll down with a rounded back.
• 3. Keep your knees slightly bent throughout the pose.

CAUTION: This pose should not be attempted without a doctor's permission by anyone suffering from glaucoma, high blood pressure, or hypertension. If this is an issue for you, you may try this variation:

• Standing comfortably erect, inhale and extend your arms out to the sides at shoulder height.

• Exhale as you slowly come forward to half way down pivoting at the hip, keeping your back flat.

• Inhale as you come up.

BENEFITS: Increases strength and flexibility of the spine and hips, lengthens hamstrings, brings increased blood supply into the head and face.

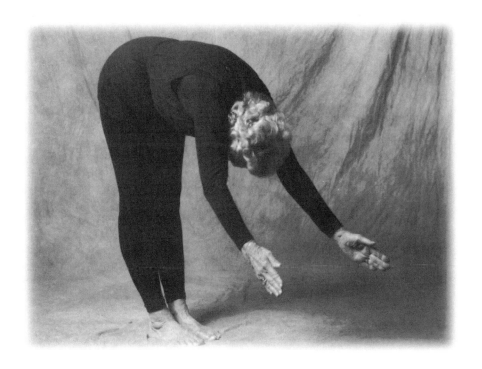

# ☜ POSE 7: ARCH ☞

*"Too much of a good thing is simply wonderful."*
—Liberace

⊡ While still in the Forward Fold, inhale as you press your chest forward and up. (If your fingers don't touch the floor you may rest your hands against your shins or thighs.)

⊡ Lengthen your spine by pressing out through the crown of your head in front of you and back through your tailbone behind you.

⊡ Inhale as you arch up, flattening your back. Exhale as you release back down into the forward fold.

BENEFITS: Strengthens the back and increases spinal flexibility, tones the legs and lengthens the hamstrings, tones the nervous system and internal organs.

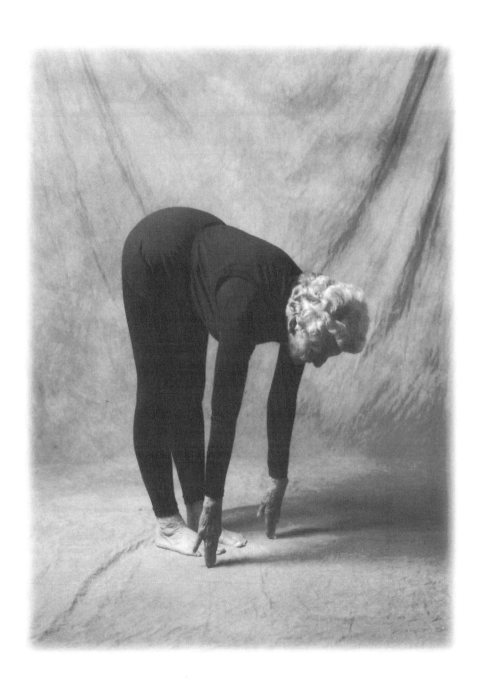

# POSE 8: LUNGE
## (Right side)

*"Do not be too squeamish and timid about your actions. All life is an experiment."*
—Ralph Waldo Emerson

⊡ Place your hands on the floor on both sides of your left foot and step back with your right foot.

⊡ As you inhale, stretch your right leg out behind you, toes pointed away and the top of the foot on the floor. Your left knee should be bent in front of you and should be supporting some of your body weight, along with your hands.

⊡ Try to lift your ribs away from your thigh as you gently stretch the right hip and thigh.

⊡ Lift through the crown of your head as you breathe deeply and evenly for 3 to 5 breaths.

⊡ Take a deep inhalation and . . .

BENEFITS: Improves posture and balance, strengthens the spine, back and legs, opens the hips, tones the arms.

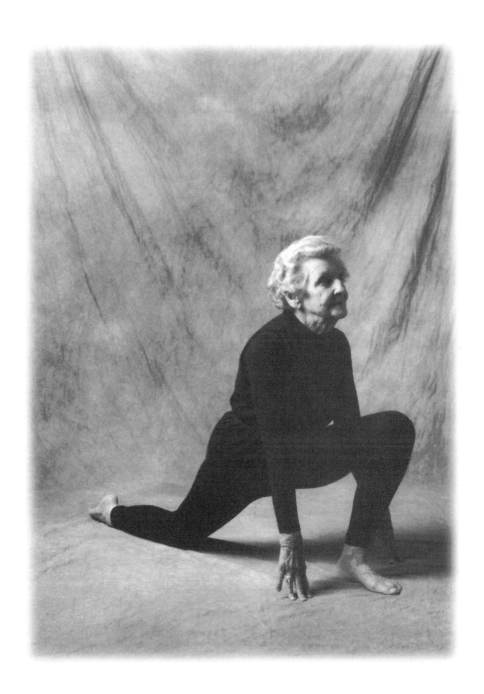

# POSE 9: DOWN DOG

*"Use your weaknesses; aspire to strength."*
—Sir Laurence Olivier

⊡ Exhale deeply as you step your left foot back beside your right foot behind you. Your body should form an upside-down "V."

⊡ Press the floor away from you with the heels of your hands as you tip your tailbone upward and press your hips back behind you.

⊡ Press your heels gently down toward the floor.

⊡ Tuck your chin softly toward your chest and try to relax your shoulders as you lengthen your arms.

⊡ Take 3 to 5 slow, steady, deep inhalations and exhalations, then . . .

NOTE: If you need to rest you may come down to your knees, bring your hips toward your heels. Remember to continue your "Ujjayi" breathing, even when resting.

CAUTION: This pose should not be attempted without a doctor's permission by anyone suffering from glaucoma, high blood pressure, or hypertension. If this is an issue for you, try this alternative:
• Bring your knees together on the floor and exhale as you lower your hips toward your heels keeping your arms stretched out on the floor in front of you.

• Let your head relax.
• As you inhale, feel your breath expand under your arms and release your lower back.

BENEFITS: Strengthens the upper body, stretches the hamstrings, strengthens the arms, legs, back and shoulders, massages abdominal organs, tones the nervous and circulatory systems.

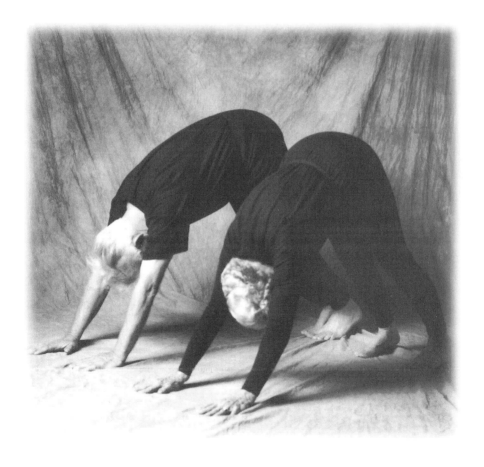

# POSE 10: LUNGE
## (Left side)

*"What keeps the body restricted is not a true physical*
*block, but a mental pattern block.*
*The blocks exist in the mind."*
—Milton Trager, M.D.

⊞ Inhaling, bring your right foot forward between your hands.

⊞ Exhale as you stretch your left leg out behind you, toes pointed away and the top of your foot on the floor.

⊞ Inhale deeply again as you lift through the crown of your head, lifting your ribs away from your right thigh.

⊞ Feel the stretch in your left thigh and right hip.

⊞ Keep breathing evenly for 3 to 5 breaths.

⊞ Inhale as you bring your right foot forward next to the left and . . .

BENEFITS: Builds strength and flexibility in the legs, thighs, back and abdomen. Improves balance, strengthens feet and ankles.

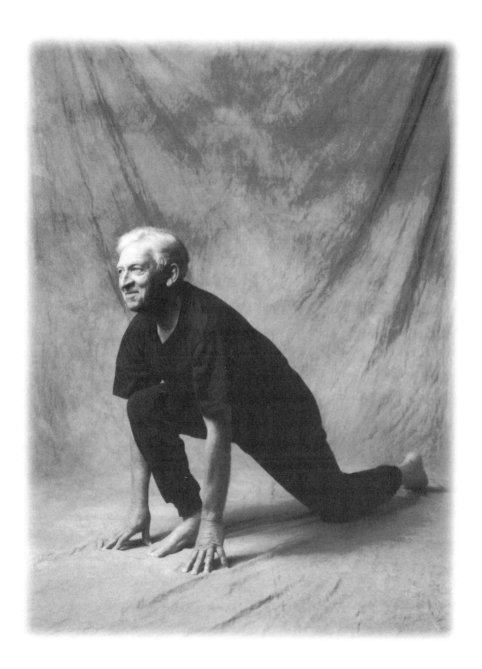

# POSE 11: FORWARD FOLD

*"You gotta have a dream, if you don't have a dream,*
*how you gonna make a dream come true?"*
—Rogers and Hammerstein

⊡ Press into the floor with both feet, lifting your tailbone toward the ceiling.

⊡ Exhale as you release your body into a Forward Fold.

⊡ Keep your knees soft and go only as far as you can keeping your knees straight.

⊡ Take 3 to 5 breaths as you tune in to releasing space between your vertebrae and relaxing downward with each exhalation.

CAUTION: This pose should not be attempted without a doctor's permission by those suffering from glaucoma, high blood pressure, or hypertension. If this is an issue for you, you may try this alternative:
• Standing comfortably erect, inhale and extend your arms out to the sides at shoulder height.
• Exhale as you slowly come forward to halfway down, pivoting the hip, keeping your back flat.
• Reach out through the crown of your head and press back behind you through your tailbone.
• Inhale as you come up.

BENEFITS: Stretches the hamstrings and the spine, firms and tones the abdominal organs and muscles, stimulates circulation and brings increased blood supply to the head.

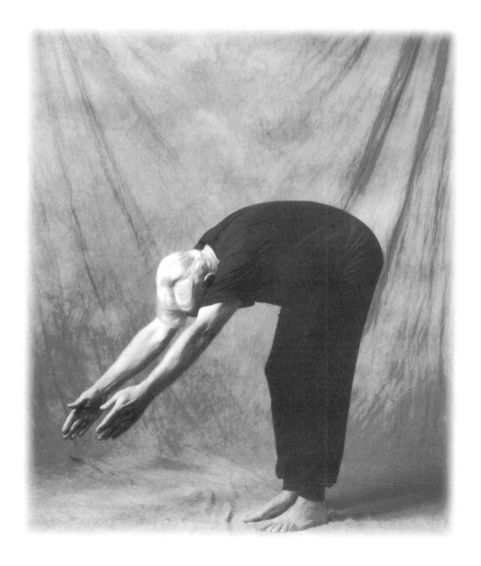

# POSE 12: DOWN DOG

*"Jonathan Seagull discovered that boredom, fear and anger are the reasons that a gull's life is so short, and with these gone from his thought, he lived a long life indeed."*
—Richard Bach

⊞ If your hands touched the floor in the previous pose, the Forward Fold, you may simply place your hands on the floor beside your feet and step your feet back behind you to bring your body into the Down Dog upside-down "V" position. Otherwise:

⊞ Bring one knee to the floor and the other down beside it.

⊞ Kneel with your knees directly below your hips and your hands directly below your shoulders.

⊞ Press your heels toward the floor and straighten your legs gently and slowly.

⊞ Lift your tailbone toward the ceiling, press the floor away from you with your hands.

⊞ Keep your chin toward your chest and your neck and shoulders relaxed as you continue to breathe deeply.

**CAUTION: This pose should not be attempted without a doctor's permission by anyone suffering from glaucoma, high blood pressure, or hypertension. If this is an issue for you, you**

may try this alternative:
• Bring yours knees to the floor and exhale as you lower your hips towards your heels.
• Keep your arms outstretched on the floor in front of you.
• As you inhale, feel the breath expand under your arms and release your lower back.

BENEFITS: Stretches the spine and hamstrings, strengthens the arms, shoulders, wrists, and hands, legs and back, massages the internal organs, increases circulation.

For a stronger practice the optional pose (C) PIGEON may be inserted here. See page 96.

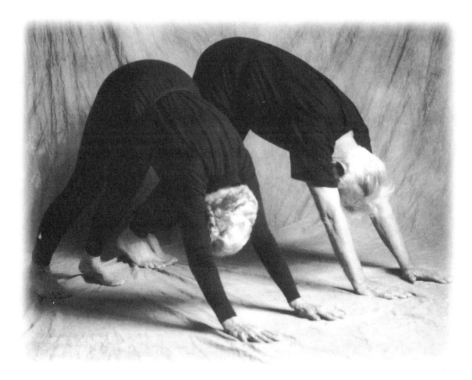

# POSE 13: CAT STRETCH

*"The most minute transformation is like a pebble dropped into a still lake. The ripples spread out endlessly."*
—Emmanuel, Pat Rodegast and Judith Stanton

⊞ Come on to your knees. Check that your knees are directly below your hips and your hands are directly below your shoulders.

⊞ Take a deep inhalation as you bend your elbows slightly and press your hands into the floor bringing your chest forward and up between your arms.

⊞ Press the crown of your head toward the ceiling and your tailbone upward, creating an exaggerated swayback.

⊞ On exhalation, arch your back upward like a Halloween cat, tucking your head and pelvic bone toward each other, pulling your bellybutton in toward your spine.

⊞ Repeat the movement several times developing a smooth, flowing rhythm combining your movement and your breath. With your fifth exhalation . . .

BENEFITS: Increases spinal flexibility, strengthens thighs, arms and shoulders, tones the abdomen, improves digestion, elimination and circulation.

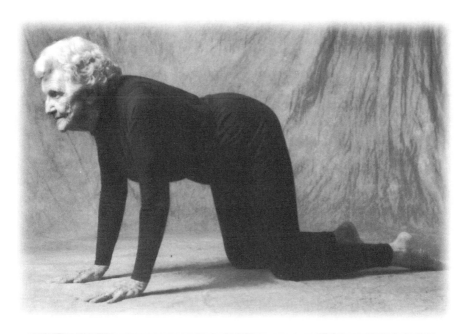

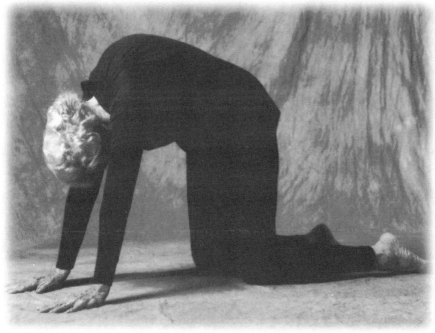

# POSE 14: EMBRYO

*"The best pay for a lovely moment is to enjoy it."*
—Richard Bach

⊡ Bring your buttocks back toward or onto your heels.

⊡ Inhale as you stretch your arms out on the floor in front of you, letting your head relax toward the floor. You may also try this pose with your arms at your sides.

⊡ Breathe deeply, trying to bring your breath down into your lower back.

⊡ Feel the stretch in your armpits and the backs of your arms.

⊡ Feel your lower back release and your vertebrae separate as you breathe deeply.

⊡ Sit up onto your heels and . . .

BENEFITS: Relaxes the spine, shoulders, and legs. Stretches the rib cage, arms, shoulders and neck. Aids in digestion, circulation, and elimination.

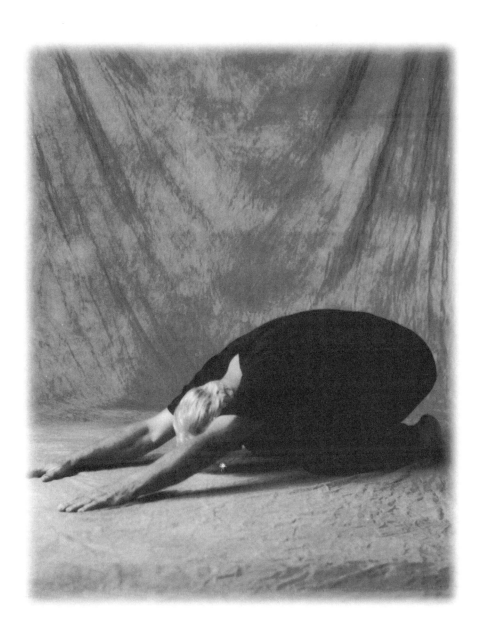

# POSE 15: COBBLER

*"The greatest discovery of my generation is that a human being
can alter his life by altering his attitudes of mind."*
—William James

⊡ Shift your left hip to the floor. Your left knee should be bent in
front of you.

⊡ Bring the soles of your feet together and let your right knee drop
out to the side.

⊡ Let your knees relax out to the sides as you gently tip your
pelvis forward pressing your bellybutton toward your heels.

⊡ Grasp your feet with your hands and carefully flatten your back,
keeping your shoulders relaxed and down.

⊡ Lift through the crown of your head.

⊡ As your flexibility increases, you may carefully walk your hands
out in front of you, letting your torso come forward. Keep your
back flat as long as you can and then gently round forward.

BENEFITS: Increases flexibility in the hips, strengthens the legs and
lower back, improves digestion and elimination.

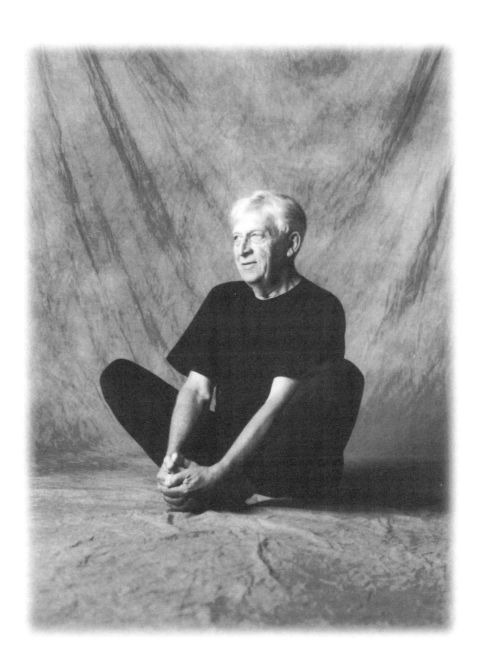

# POSE 16: SEATED HALF FORWARD FOLD
## (Right side)

*"You can't build a reputation on what you're going to do."*
—Henry Ford

⊞ Extend your right leg out in front of you keeping your left foot pressing lightly against the inside of your right thigh.

⊞ Check that both hips are facing forward and that you are sitting squarely on your "sit-bones."

⊞ Maintaining a flat back, take a deep inhalation as you raise your arms overhead, palms facing each other.

⊞ With your next inhalation, lift out of your sit-bones and stretch up through the length of your torso, out through your fingertips.

⊞ Press out through the heel of your extended foot, keeping your foot energized.

⊞ Exhale slowly, coming forward carefully, leading with your breastbone, arms extended toward your outstretched foot.

⊞ Let your hands grasp your knee, your calf or your foot, wherever they naturally come to rest without stress.

⊞ Remember to listen to the rhythm of your breathing, allowing your body to relax into the pose.

✦ With each inhalation feel your body extend a bit farther and feel it release little by little with every exhalation.

✦ Take 5 or more long, slow, even inhalations and exhalations.

✦ Bring your arms overhead and inhale as you come up with a flat back. Or you may roll up slowly inhaling, allowing your hands to slide up your leg as you curl up to a seated position.

✦ Exhale completely . . .

BENEFITS: Nourishes the spinal nerves and discs, stretches the hamstrings and ligaments of the back, tones abdominal organs, stimulates digestion and elimination.

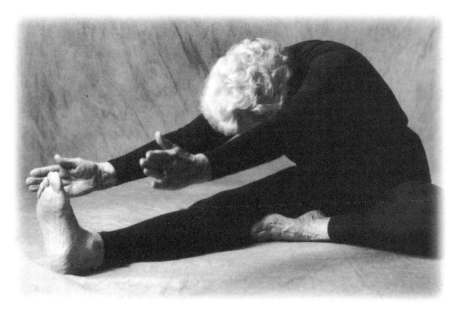

# POSE 17: NOBILITY POSE
## (Right)

*"Things won are done; joy's soul lies in the doing."*
—Shakespeare

⊡ Keeping your left knee bent, bring your right leg over your left.

⊡ Bend your right knee and bring it across the left so that one knee is above the other.

⊡ Be sure that your heels are not under your hips.

⊡ Lift your torso out of your hips, flatten your back, lift through the crown of your head.

⊡ Let your hands rest on the soles of your feet or your knees and assume an air of nobility.

⊡ If this pose is too much of a stretch you may simply cross your left ankle over your right knee and gently allow your left knee to drop out to the side.

⊡ Feel the stretch in your hips as you breathe deeply for 3 to 5 breaths. Then . . .

BENEFITS: Releases and strengthens the hips and lower back, stretches the ankles, opens the chest, relaxes the shoulders.

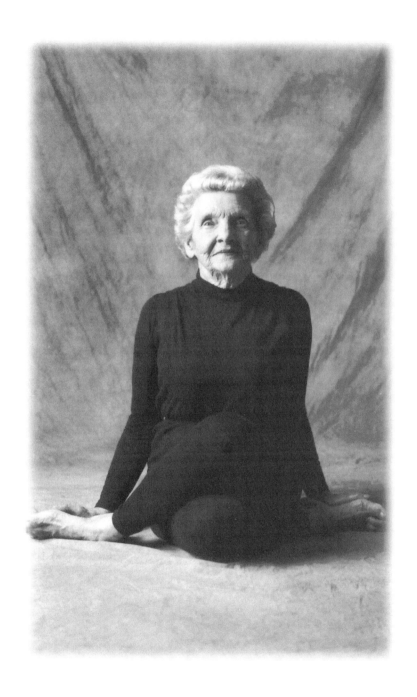

# POSE 18: SEATED SPINAL TWIST
## (Right)

*"Stop chattering, go within."*
—Sananda

⊞ Place your right foot on the floor to the outside of your left thigh.

⊞ Take a deep inhalation as you bring your left arm out to the side, shoulder height, parallel to the floor.

⊞ Exhale as you bring it around your bent right knee, resting your knee in the crook of your elbow.

⊞ Inhale as you flatten your back and raise your right arm up and overhead, lifting out of your hips and lengthening your spine.

⊞ Exhaling, lower your right hand to the floor behind you, as close to your tailbone as possible.

⊞ Inhale as you lift through the crown of your head and exhale as you rotate your chin to face over your right shoulder.

⊞ Feel your spine lengthening with each inhalation and gently twist with each exhalation, using your front arm and leg as a point of leverage.

⊞ Take 3 to 5 long slow inhalations and exhalations.

⊕ Come out of the pose gently.

⊕ Inhale as you raise your right arm up overhead and exhale as you bring your body around to face forward again, lowering your arm.

BENEFITS: Lubricates and nourishes the spinal column, promotes circulation through the internal organs improving digestion and elimination.

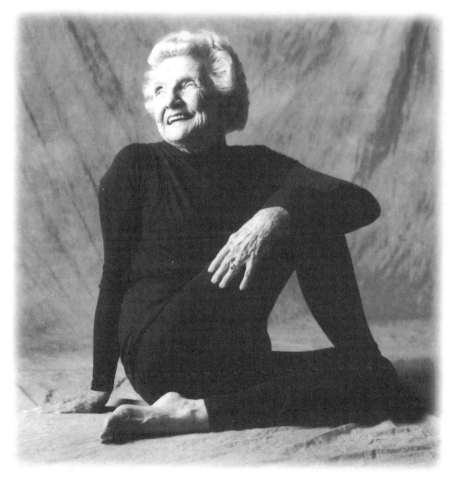

# POSE 19: SEATED FULL FORWARD FOLD

*"You create your own reality every moment of your day."*
—Shirley MacLaine

⊞ Extend both legs out in front of you.

⊞ Press out through your heels in front and through your tailbone behind you.

⊞ Inhaling, raise both arms up and overhead, palms facing each other. Stretch up, separating your ribs, lengthening your waist.

⊞ Exhale as you gently come forward keeping your arms alongside your ears, leading with your chest.

⊞ Release your arms forward and let your hands come to rest on your legs, ankles or feet. Breathe deeply for 5 or more breaths.

⊞ Relax into the pose, allow your body to slowly release tightness and soften with each exhalation.

⊞ Come up slowly, inhaling, sliding your hands along the tops of your legs.

⊞ Keep your left leg out in front of you and . . .

BENEFITS: Stretches the back and hamstrings, increases circulation in the spine, stimulates entire abdominal area as well as organs of digestion, elimination, and reproduction.

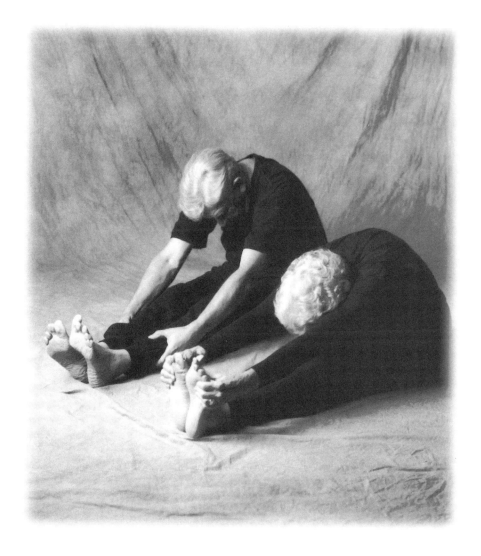

# POSE 20: SEATED HALF FORWARD FOLD
## (Left)

*"All you can do is live as if your life depended on it.
And watch what happens next."*
—Stephen Kravette

⊡ Bring your right foot in to press lightly against the inside of your left thigh.

⊡ Be sure that your hips are facing squarely forward and that you are sitting up on your "sit-bones."

⊡ Take a deep inhalation and raise your arms up overhead, lifting up and out through your fingertips.

⊡ Keep your extended foot active, pressing out through your heel.

⊡ Exhale as you come forward slowly, keeping your back flat, arms extended out in front of you.

⊡ Release your arms to their natural resting place without stress on your lower back.

⊡ Listen to the rhythm of your breathing and relax into the pose.

⊡ Feel your body open up as you inhale and feel it release as you exhale.

✛ Take 5 or more strong yet gentle inhalations and exhalations.

✛ Inhaling, come up with arms overhead or curl up slowly to a seated position.

✛ Exhale completely.

✛ Keep your right knee bent as you . . .

BENEFITS: Increases circulation in the nerves, discs, and muscles of the spine, massages the internal organs, stimulates digestion and elimination.

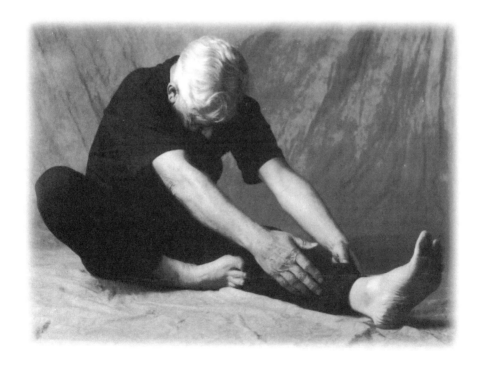

# POSE 21: NOBILITY POSE
## (Left)

*"The first secret you should know about perfect health*
*is that you have to choose it."*
—Deepak Chopra, M.D.

⊡ Bring your left leg over your right.

⊡ Bend your left knee and bring it around so that one knee is above the other.

⊡ Press your sit-bones into the floor, relax your shoulders and extend through the crown of your head.

⊡ Try to maintain a strong, flat back and let your hands rest on the soles of your feet.

⊡ Feel the stretch in your hips as you lift your chest and expand your ribcage.

⊡ If this stretch is too challenging, you may cross your right ankle over your left knee and allow your right knee to gently fall out to the side.

⊡ Breathe deeply for 3 to 5 breaths.

⊡ Then . . .

BENEFITS: Increases hip flexibility and strengthens lower back, stretches outer thighs, knees and ankles, opens the chest, relaxes the shoulders.

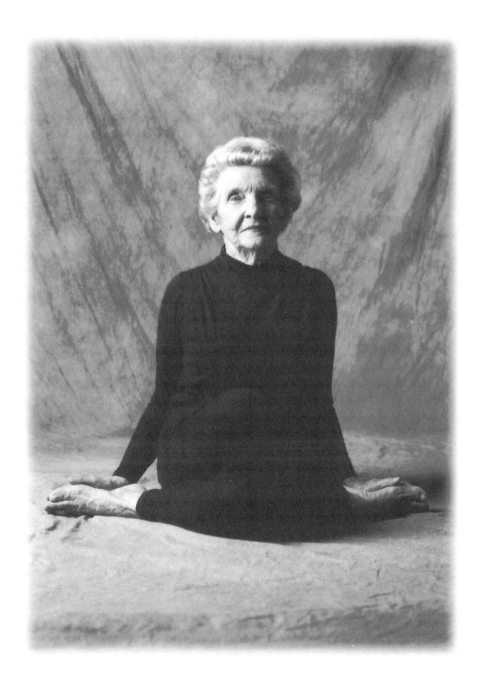

# POSE 22: SEATED SPINAL TWIST
## (Left)

*"Don't let life discourage you; everyone who got
where he is had to begin where he was."*
—Richard L. Evans

⊡ Place your left foot on the floor to the outside of your right thigh.

⊡ Inhale deeply as you extend your right arm out to the side, shoulder height, parallel to the floor.

⊡ Exhaling, bring it around your bent left knee, holding your knee with the inside of your elbow.

⊡ Inhale as you raise your left arm up and overhead.

⊡ Exhaling, lower your left hand to the floor behind you, as close to your spine as you can. Press your hand into the floor, flattening your back.

⊡ Be sure that both sit bones stay squarely on the floor.

⊡ Inhale as you lift through the crown of your head and exhale as you rotate your chin to face over your left shoulder.

⊡ Press against the floor to lengthen your spine with each inhalation and gently twist with each exhalation, using your front arm and leg as a point of leverage.

⊡ Take 3 to 5 long slow inhalations and exhalations.

⊡ Come out of the pose gently. Inhaling as you raise your left arm up overhead and exhaling as you bring your body around to face forward again, lowering your arm.

BENEFITS: Increases elasticity of the muscles and ligaments of the spine, can prevent backache, massages internal organs toning liver, kidneys and spleen. Aids digestion and elimination.

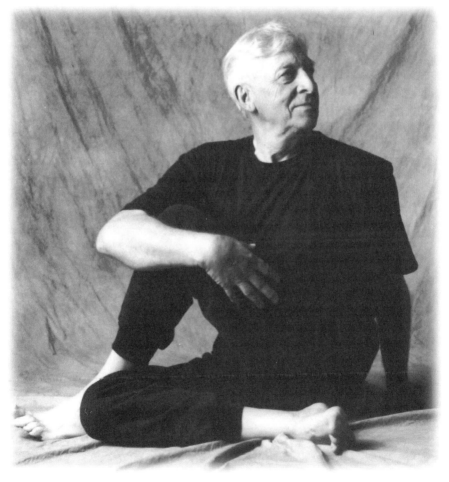

# POSE 23: UPWARD FACING BOAT

*"There's only one corner of the universe you can be certain of improving and that's your own self."*
—Aldous Huxley

⊡ Bring both legs in front of you, knees bent, toes on the floor.

⊡ Grasp your legs behind your knees, inhale as you press your ribs toward your thighs, flattening your back.

⊡ Exhale as you round your back, pressing out behind you through your waist.

⊡ Inhale as you press your ribs toward your thighs again.

⊡ Find your balance point as you tip back slightly on your sit-bones, slowly letting your toes leave the floor and raising your shins.

⊡ Take a deep inhalation and exhale as you press out through the balls of your feet extending them out in front of you.

⊡ Keep your shoulders relaxed and arms extended, either holding behind your knees or your arms outstretched beside them.

⊡ Keep your chest lifted and feel your abdominal and thigh muscles supporting you.

⊡ Maintain your deep breathing as you hold the pose for 3 to 5 breaths.

✦ Bring your toes back to the floor and . . .

BENEFITS: Develops balance and strengthens abdominal muscles, thighs, hips and back. Tones the nervous system.

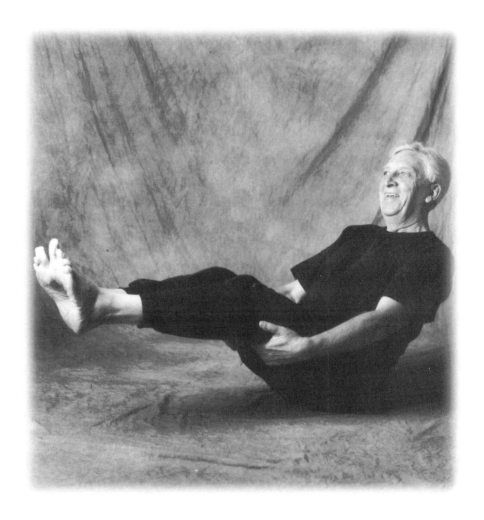

# POSE 24: KNEE CIRCLES

*"I take care of me. I'm the only one I've got."*
—Groucho Marx

⊡ Gently and slowly roll yourself back to the floor one vertebrae at a time.

⊡ Pull your knees into your chest.

⊡ Place one hand on each knee and make circles with your knees together, first clockwise, then counter clockwise.

⊡ Smaller circles massage your lower back close to the spine and larger circles massage outward toward the hips.

⊡ Experiment to see what feels the best and enjoy your self-massage.

⊡ Be conscious of your breathing rhythm.

⊡ Slide your legs out in front of you and . . .

BENEFITS: Resting posture, relieves lower back strain, massages abdominal wall and intestines, relieves indigestion and gas pressure.

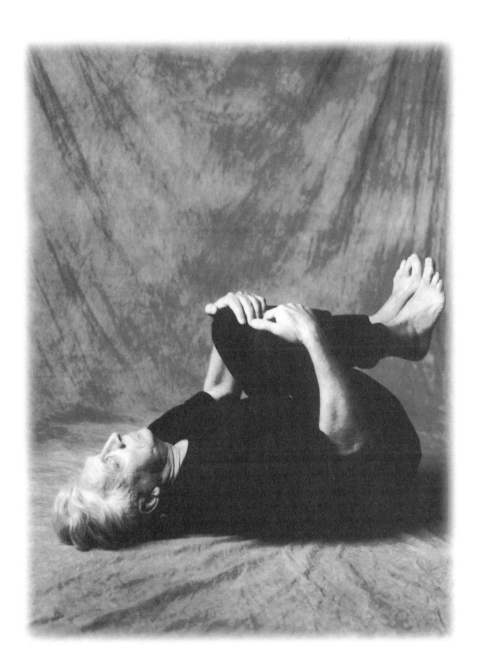

# POSE 25: LYING SPINAL TWIST
## (Right)

*"Flow with whatever may happen and let your mind be free;*
*stay centered by accepting whatever you are doing."*
—Chuang Tzu

⊞ Extend your arms out to your sides at shoulder height, palms facing the floor.

⊞ Bending your left knee, bring your left foot to rest on top of your right knee or shin.

⊞ Take a deep inhalation and press out through the heel of your extended right foot.

⊞ Exhale as you lower your left knee across to your right side, bringing your right hand to gently press your left knee toward the floor.

⊞ Try to keep your left shoulder touching the floor.

⊞ Inhale as you rotate your head to look toward your left hand.

⊞ Exhale as you release your body into the pose.

⊞ Continue your breathing for 3 to 5 breaths, pressing out through your extended foot and releasing your knee toward the floor.

⊞ Take a deep inhalation and bring your left knee to your chest.

⊞ Exhale as you roll back onto your back, and . . .

BENEFITS: Massages internal organs, stretches ligaments and muscles of the spine, increases spinal flexibility, hydrates and nourishes spinal discs.

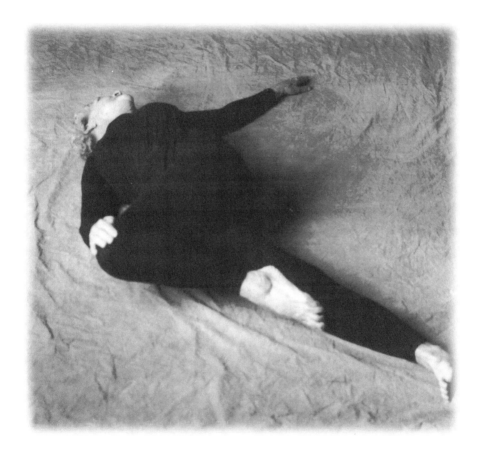

# POSE 26: LEG RAISES
## (Right)

*"There is nothing permanent except change."*
—Heraclitus

⊡ Holding your left knee in toward your chest, press out through the heel of your extended right foot.

⊡ Inhale as you raise your right leg up toward the ceiling, pointing your toes.

⊡ Keep your leg as straight as possible. If you feel any stress on your lower back, bend your knee.

⊡ Flex your foot and exhale as you slowly lower your leg toward the floor.

⊡ Point your toes and inhale, raising your leg.

⊡ Flex your foot and exhale, lowering your leg.

⊡ Continue for 3 to 5 repetitions, then bring both knees into your chest.

NOTE: If you would like more of a challenge, you may hold your extended foot a few inches above the floor for a breath before raising your leg.

BENEFITS: Strengthens the abdominal and lower back muscles, tones the legs and hips.

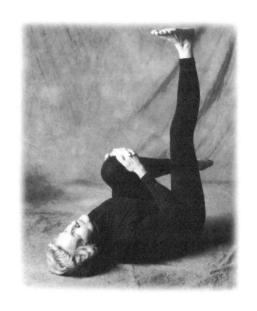

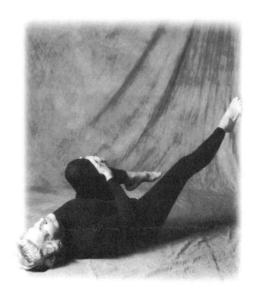

# POSE 27: LYING SPINAL TWIST
## (Left)

*"A man consists of the faith that is in him. Whatever his faith, he is."*
—The Bhagavad-Gita

⊡ Extend your left leg out in front of you and your arms out to your sides at shoulder height.

⊡ This time bend your right knee, bringing your right foot to rest on top of your left knee or leg.

⊡ Inhale as you press out through the heel of your extended left leg.

⊡ Exhaling, lower your right knee across to the left, press your left hand gently on your right knee.

⊡ Keep your right shoulder pressing toward the floor.

⊡ Inhale and turn your head to look over your left shoulder.

⊡ Exhale and relax into the pose.

⊡ Breathe evenly for 3 to 5 breaths, keeping your extended foot flexed.

⊡ Mentally direct your breath into resistant areas of your body.

⊡ Inhale as you bring your right knee to your chest.

⊡ Exhale as you roll back to center, and . . .

BENEFITS: Stretches, tones and hydrates the spinal discs and ligaments, massages internal organs, increases flexibility of spine, back and ribs.

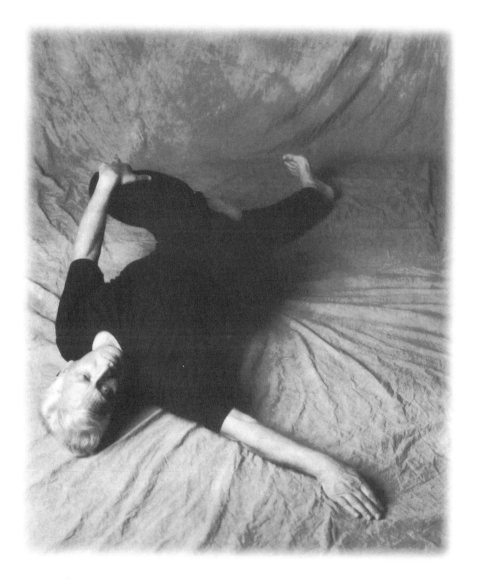

# POSE 28: LEG RAISES
## (Left)

*"Do not look at your body as a stranger, but adopt a friendly approach towards it. To be sensitive is to be alive."*
—Vanda Scaravelli

⊡ Hold your right knee in toward your chest and extend your left leg, pointing your toes.

⊡ Flex your foot and exhale, slowly lowering your leg to the floor.

⊡ Inhale and raise your left leg upward keeping your toes pointed and your knee as straight as possible.

⊡ Flex your foot and exhale, extending out through your heel as you lower your leg.

⊡ Point your toes and inhale, raising your leg.

⊡ Continue for 3 to 5 repetitions, then bring both knees into your chest.

BENEFITS: Strengthens the abdominal and lower back muscles, tones the legs and hips.

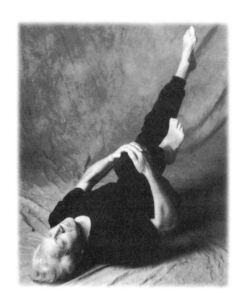

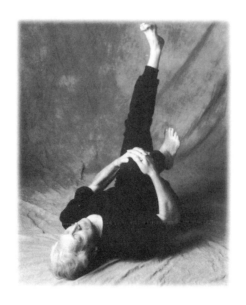

# POSE 29: KNEE CIRCLES

*"Life just is.*
*You have to flow with it.*
*Give yourself to the moment. Let it happen."*
—Jerry Brown

⊡ With your knees tucked into your chest, circle your knees to massage and relax your lower back.

⊡ Circle clockwise, then counter clockwise.

⊡ Breathe into your lower back as you release tension and increase circulation.

BENEFITS: Relieves lower back tension, massages lower back muscles and intestines, relieves indigestion and gas pressure.

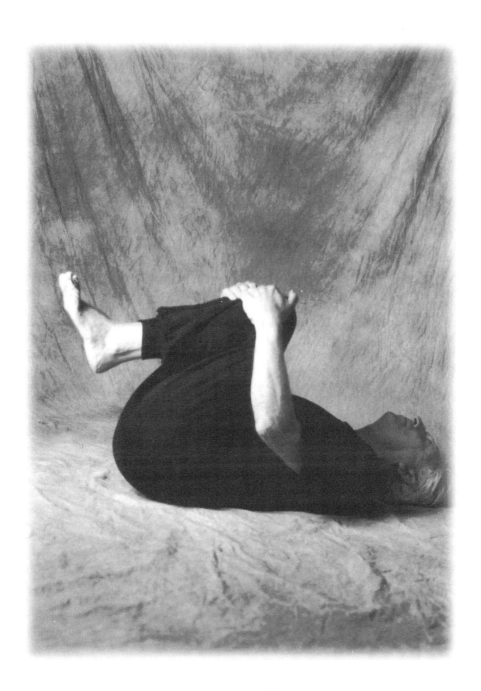

# POSE 30: BRIDGE

*"It does not matter how slowly you go so long as you do not stop."*
—Confucius

⊞ Place your feet on the floor just in front of your buttocks.

⊞ Let your arms rest by your sides, palms down.

⊞ Press the back of your waist into the floor and tip your tailbone under and up.

⊞ Inhale as you press into the floor with your feet and raise your pelvis upward, keeping your tail tucked under.

⊞ Breathe deeply and steadily, holding the pose for 3 to 5 breaths.

⊞ Feel your buttocks supporting you from behind and your thighs holding the lift.

⊞ Take a deep inhalation and come up onto your toes.

⊞ Exhale as you slowly roll down, one vertebrae at a time, keeping your back rounded, your tailbone should touch the floor last.

**CAUTION: This pose should not be attempted without a doctor's permission by anyone suffering from glaucoma, high blood pressure, or hypertension. If this is an issue for you, you may want to skip this pose.**

BENEFITS: Strengthens the buttocks, legs, neck and spine, brings fresh blood to the head, opens the chest, stimulates the pineal, pituitary and thyroid glands.

Optional pose: (D), LEGS UP THE WALL, may be inserted here. See page 98.

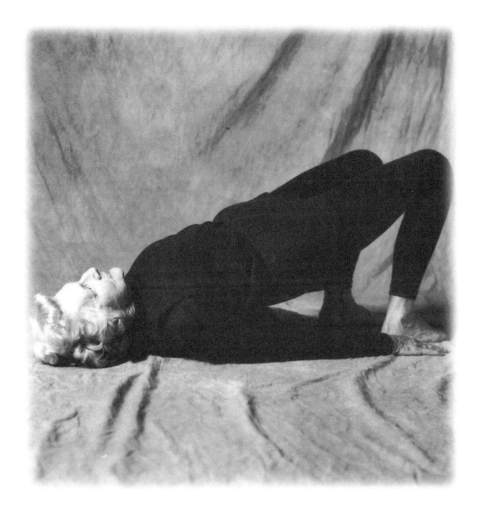

# POSE 31: PRANAYAMA
## (Controlled breathing)

*"One is one's present self, what one was and
what one will become, all at once."*
—Peter Matthiessen

**CAUTION: Controlled breathing techniques should not be attempted without a doctor's permission by anyone suffering from glaucoma, high blood pressure, or hypertension. If this is an issue for you, you may want to skip this pose.**

⊞ Stretch your legs out on the floor in front of you and release your body to the floor.

⊞ Take a long, slow, relaxed inhalation while counting silently to 5.

⊞ Fill your lungs completely, feeling your ribs expand and your diaphragm drop. Gently hold the air in for several counts.

⊞ Exhale with control to the count of 5, feeling your diaphragm lift and squeezing all the air out of your lungs.

⊞ Repeat for 3 to 5 inhalations and exhalations.

⊞ Let your body resume its normal breathing rhythm.

NOTE: If it is too much of a challenge to breathe to the count of 5, begin your breathing practice with counts of 2 or 3 and build up your breath control gradually. Conversely, if breathing to the count of 5 is not challenging for you, increase your breath count gradually to build up your lung capacity and muscle control.

BENEFITS: Develops muscle control, increases lung capacity, produces a state of tranquillity, quiets the mind and oxygenates the body.

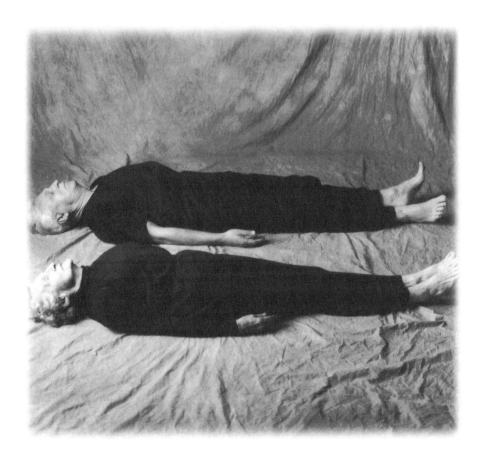

# POSE 32: SAVASANA
## (Deep relaxation)

*"My life has no purpose, no direction, no aim, no meaning,*
*and yet I'm happy. I can't figure it out.*
*What am I doing right?"*
—Charles M. Schulz

⊡ Release your entire body to the support of the floor, arms by your sides, palms facing up.

⊡ Visualize each part of your body letting go as you mentally scan your body from your toes up through the top of your head.

⊡ Tell yourself to relax your feet and ankles, relax your calves and the backs of your knees. Release your lower back and so on up to your jaw, brow, scalp and the crown of your head.

⊡ Allow about 10 minutes for relaxation. This is an important time for the body to balance itself, gather energy, and integrate the benefits of your practice.

⊡ It is important to come out of the relaxation pose very slowly to avoid dizziness or light-headedness. Begin by bringing your knees to your chest and resting for a moment, then roll over to your right side and remain in the fetal position for 2 or 3 breaths.

⊡ Slowly push yourself up into a comfortable seated posture, eyes closed, and take 5 long, deep inhalations and exhalations.

⊡ Thank your body for its service to you and thank yourself for caring for your body.

BENEFITS: Balances the benefits of your practice, completes relaxation, quiets the mind, reduces fatigue, rejuvenates the body and mind.

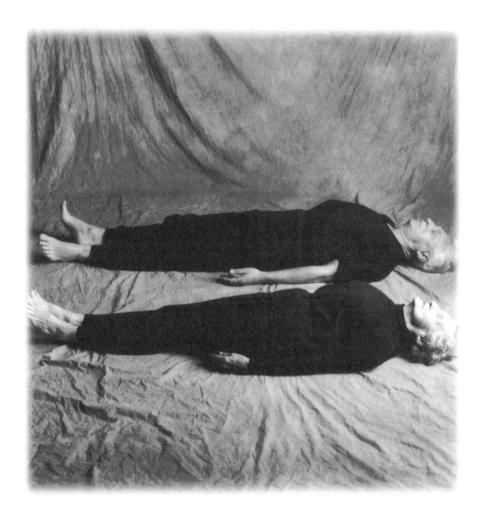

# OPTIONAL POSES

## (More challenging)

# POSE A: TREE

*"Do what you can with what you have where you are."*
—Theodore Roosevelt

⊡ Stand squarely on both feet, lifting through the crown of the head.

⊡ Fix your gaze on a point in front of you.

⊡ Place your right hand on your hip and inhale as you raise your left arm out to the side and overhead.

⊡ Bring your right foot to the inside of your left calf, your knee out to the side.

⊡ Breathe evenly, lifting through the crown of your head as you inhale and pressing your standing foot into the floor as you exhale. Be sure to keep your tail tucked under to avoid unnecessary stress on the lower back.

⊡ Repeat the pose on the opposite side:

⊡ Raise your right arm out to the side and overhead.

⊡ Standing on your right leg, bring your left foot to your right calf.

⊡ As you become more proficient in balancing, you may position your foot higher and higher on your standing leg.

NOTE: If balancing is challenging for you, you may begin practicing this pose with your hands on your hips, and gradually raise your arm as you become more proficient.

BENEFITS: Develops balance, concentration and poise, strengthens buttocks, lower back, legs, feet, and ankles. Stretches ribs, shoulders, and arms.

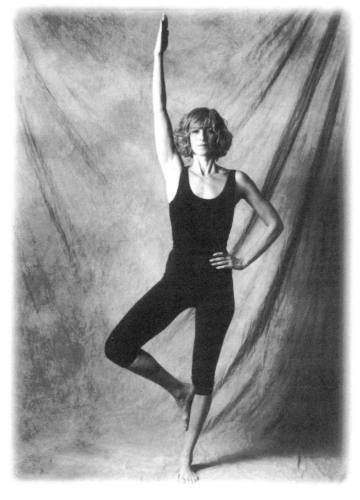

# POSE B: TRIANGLE

*"There is no failure except in no longer trying."*
—Elbert Hubbard

⊡ Step your right foot forward approximately three feet.

⊡ Turn your back foot to a 90° angle, letting a line from the heel of your front foot bisect the arch of your back foot.

⊡ Inhale as you raise your arms out to the sides making sure that your hips are facing forward.

⊡ Shift your back hip toward your back heel and reach out over your front foot with your front hand.

⊡ Exhale as you lower your torso to the side, bringing your front arm toward your shin and raising your back arm up toward the ceiling.

⊡ You may turn your head to look up at your raised hand or look down at your forward foot.

⊡ Breathe deeply, reaching your raised arm upward and extending forward through the crown of your head and back through your tailbone.

⊡ Hold the pose and breathe, 3 to 5 breaths.

⊡ Repeat on the opposite side.

BENEFITS: Lengthens hamstrings, increases flexibility of the hips and spine, firms legs and waist, stretches arms shoulders and back, opens the chest, nourishes the abdominal organs and spine.

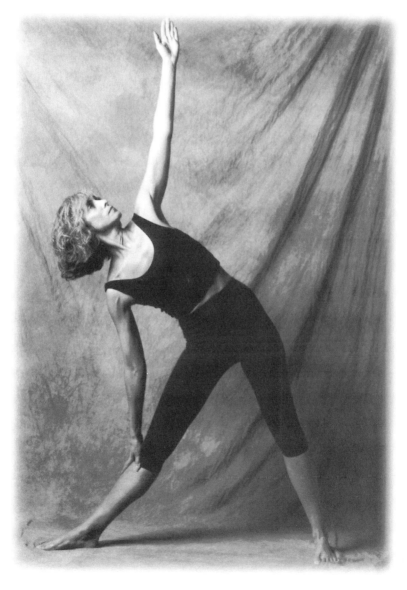

# POSE C: PIGEON

*"Even if you're on the right track
you'll get run over if you just sit there.*
—Will Rogers

Transitioning from the Down Dog position (Pose 12, Page 48):

⊡ Lay your forward leg across in front of your torso, knee out to the side.

⊡ Stretch your back leg out behind you, as in the Lunge, top of the foot on the floor and toes pointing away.

⊡ Press your hands into the floor in front of you and inhale. Lift your chest and arch your back slightly, lifting through the crown of your head.

⊡ Breathe evenly, long, deep inhalations and exhalations for 3 to 5 breaths.

⊡ Turn the toes of your back foot under and step your front foot back into the Down Dog, pressing the floor away from you with your hands.

⊡ Take several breaths in the Down Dog—full inhalations and complete exhalations.

⊡ Bring the opposite leg forward to repeat the pose on the opposite side.

BENEFITS: Increases flexibility in the hips, strengthens the back, opens the chest.

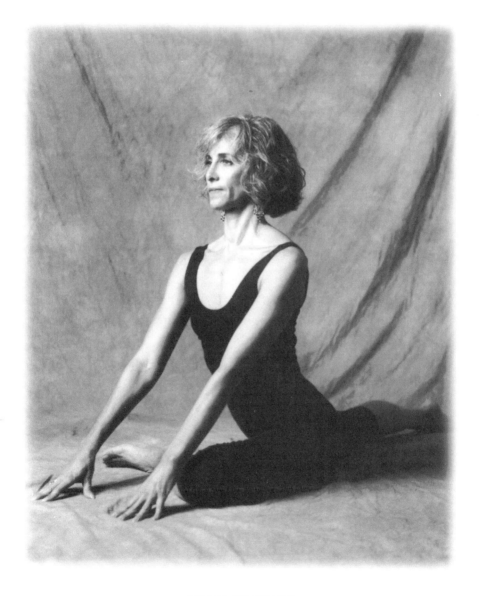

# ≡ POSE D: LEGS UP THE WALL ⌐

*"May you live all the days of your life."*
—Jonathan Swift

⊡ Sit sideways with one hip against a wall.

⊡ Lie back carefully and rotate your body so that you can bring your legs up the wall perpendicular to your torso.

⊡ Keep your breath strong and rhythmic.

⊡ Maintain this posture for 5 to 10 minutes. If this seems like too much, begin with 2 to 3 minutes and gradually increase the time.

⊡ Bring your knees to your chest and take several breaths. Then roll over to one side and swivel around so that you can extend your legs out in front of you.

NOTE: Take your time getting up to avoid dizziness.

**CAUTION: This pose should not be attempted without a doctor's permission by anyone suffering from glaucoma, high blood pressure, or hypertension. If this is an issue for you, you may want to skip this pose.**

BENEFITS: Stretches and firms legs, beneficial for varicose veins and circulation, relieves tension in the hips, relaxes the lower back.

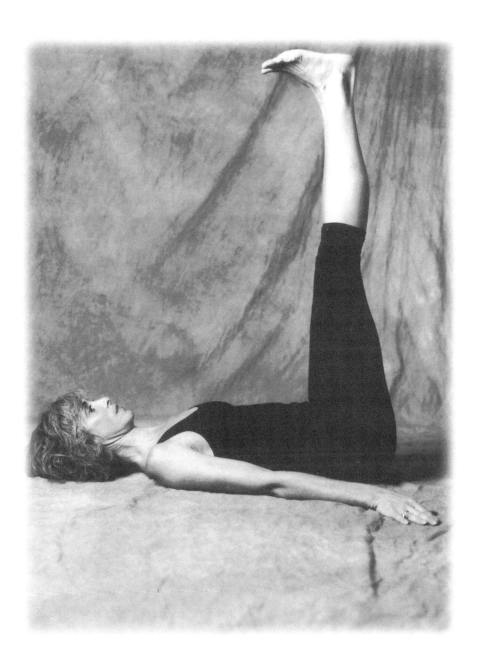

# BIBLIOGRAPHY AND SUGGESTED READING

Barnard, Neal. *Food for Life*. New York: Harmony Books, 1993.

Bell, Lorna and Seyfer, Eudora. *Gentle Yoga*. Berkeley, CA: Celestial Arts, 1982.

Chopra, Deepak. *Ageless Body, Timeless Mind: The Quantum Alternative to Growing Old*. New York: Harmony Books, 1993.

Hewitt, James. *The Complete Yoga Book*. New York: Schocken Books, 1977.

Kravette, Stephen. *Alternatives to Aging*. West Chester, PA: Whitford Press, 1989.

Null, Gary. *Reverse the Aging Process*. New York: Villard Books, Random House, 1993.

Ornish, Dean. *Reversing Heart Disease*. New York: Random House, 1990.

Paul, Stephen C. *Inneractions*. New York: Harper-Collins, 1992.

Robbins, John. *Diet for a New America*. Walpole, NH: Stillpoint Publishing, 1987.

Samskrti and Veda. *Hatha Yoga, Manual I*. The Himalayan International Institute of Yoga Science and Philosophy, 1977.

Scaravelli, Vanda. *Awakening the Spine*. San Francisco: Harper, 1991.

Trager, Milton. *Trager Mentastics*. Barrytown, NY: Station Hill Press, 1987.

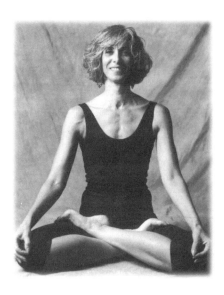
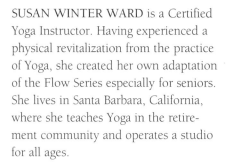
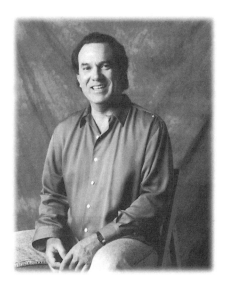

SUSAN WINTER WARD is a Certified Yoga Instructor. Having experienced a physical revitalization from the practice of Yoga, she created her own adaptation of the Flow Series especially for seniors. She lives in Santa Barbara, California, where she teaches Yoga in the retirement community and operates a studio for all ages.

JOHN SIROIS entered the world of photography when he was eight, capturing his many siblings with a Kodak Brownie Hawkeye. Today he still loves to photograph people, although his cameras are a bit more sophisticated, such as the 4X5 Gowland twin reflex he used to shoot the photos for this book. John is a "Baby Boomer," originally from Massachusetts, now residing in Santa Barbara.

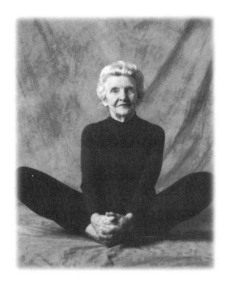 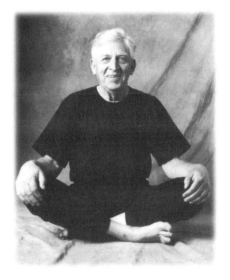

BABS RAYMOND is a widow with three daughters and six grandchildren. She has lived in the Samarkand Retirement Community for six years, where she joined Susan Ward's Yoga class which she describes as "entirely uplifting."

OTTO MORTENSEN, an architect, came to America from Copenhagen thirty-seven years ago. Now retired and living in Santa Barbara, he's been a Yoga enthusiast for more than twenty years and is the proud patriarch of a son and daughter, and two grandchildren.

# Your Personal Exercise Schedule

# Your Personal Exercise Schedule

# Your Personal Exercise Schedule

# Your Personal Exercise Schedule

# Your Personal Exercise Schedule

# Your Personal Exercise Schedule

# Your Personal Exercise Schedule

# Your Personal Exercise Schedule